**Homema**

MW01114010

# TOP 30 Effective Natural Remedies and Best

# Organic Recipes for Healing Without Pills

# Table of content:

## Introduction - Antibiotics...

They seem to be the go-to prescription when you have a virus or infection, but taking them can leave you with other problems that will need correcting, like candida or digestive disorders. You take to the internet to find information on natural alternatives to the antibiotics your doctor prescribes. The problem is the searches leave you either with more questions or conflicting information. You are in luck, this book was written to give you the knowledge in an easy-to-understand format without leaving you with more questions. So if you are ready to take charge of your health and learn about all natural recommendations, this book is right up your alley!

# Chapter 1 - Your Immune System

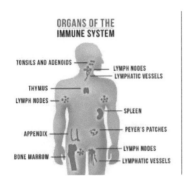

Out of all the systems your body has, the immune is the one that is on the front lines fighting colds, viruses, and infections. It works in conjunction with your other systems to keep you healthy and running on all cylinders. To better care for your immune system, you have to get to know your immune system.

*Tonsils*

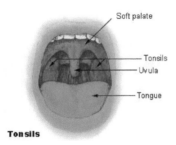

**Tonsils**

These are your first line of defense in your immune system. They help protect your body from any pathogens that try to enter from your nose and mouth. They are top notch at doing this, but sometimes they need to be extracted when they are constantly becoming infected due to bacteria.

## Lymph Nodes

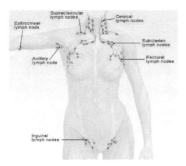

Located throughout your body, they are the filters of waste, and conveyors of nutrients and lymph fluids to different parts of your body. Your lymph nodes are one of the most important parts of your immune system. When they are overtaxed due to illnesses, they tend to swell, and in more severe cases, be the target of cancer.

## The Thymus

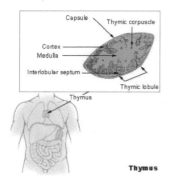

Though many would put this gland with another body system, it is closely related to the lymph nodes in the immune system. It play a key role in the manufacture of T-lymphocytes (T Cells), one of the more important types of white blood cells. It gets immature white blood cells from the bone marrow and teaches them how to attack foreign cells, like bacteria and viruses, in the body.

*The Spleen*

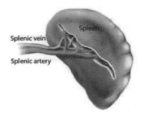

This part of the immune system recycles red blood cells and platelets. It also serves as a storage space for white blood cells. The spleen also plays a part in fight the bacteria that can lead to pneumonia and meningitis. When this organ becomes enlarged, it is due to mononucleosis, some diseases of the liver, and some cancers. When it is ruptured because of an accident, it causes internal bleeding that can be life-threatening.

*The Appendix*

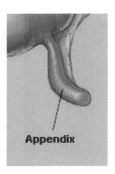

Even though it is attached to the colon, it actually plays a part in the immune system. The appendix has lymphatic vessels and can play a role in fighting off pathogens and bacteria. Current studies say that it may play a large roll in preventing the more serious diseases. When it is taxed to the limit, it can swell an rupture, leading to its removal.

*Peyer's Patches*

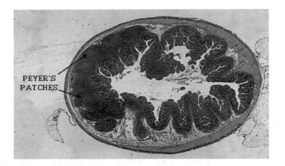

These are found in different places in the small intestine. It keeps an eye on intestinal bacteria populations and can help to stop the growth of those bacteria which can turn into pathogens. They are little egg-shaped patches of tissue.

*Bone Marrow*

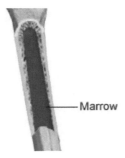

This is the spongy tissue found in the center of the bones. They convey oxygen to many parts of your body and are also responsible for the manufacture of the white blood cells which go to the Thymus to be trained. Marrow also contains stem cells and platelets which help with clotting. White blood cells combat foreign invaders in your body, such as infections and viruses.

*Causes for Immune System Weakness*

Our immune system works around the clock and can prevent illnesses when you take care of yourself. However, poor diet, poor quality and quantity of sleep, adverse changes in weather, and constantly being under stress can lead to your immune system being compromised, making you feel tired and also increasing your susceptibility to getting sick.

## Poor Diet

In this society of constantly running around and wanting things done as soon as possible, our choices for healthy food have turned into going to the local drive-through to pick up a burger and fries. Doing so every once in a while is not bad, like anything in moderation, but eating fast foods and highly processed food deprives your body of the vital nutrients your body needs on a daily basis to keep your immune system functioning properly.

A little preparation goes a long way in this area. Plan your meals for the week and package them, including healthy snacks. There are food storage options that make this easier than it used to be to prepare full meals and store them for quick meals. There are also healthy meals that can be prepared in less than 15 minutes to make cooking convenient and not time consuming. In the most rushed settings, a good vitamin packed protein shake can work in a pinch as well.

## Poor Sleep Habits

On average, a body needs six to eight hours of sleep to be feel refreshed and give your immune a chance to do its job. The immune system does its best work when you are asleep, where it uses your energy while sleeping to speed healing and fight colds. If you find it hard to sleep at night, try turning off your phone and computer an hour before bed. This includes your tablet.

Give your brain time to rest from the stimuli of constant internet searches, texting, and checking your social media notifications. When your mind has time to rest, your body will often follow suit. Don't go to bed while you are still thinking about something. Your mind will try to come up with a solution to the problem you go to bed having. Write it down and then try sleeping.

## Changes in the Weather

We can't control the weather, but we can control how we prepare for it. Take those extra few minutes to check the weather and plan accordingly. Always keep an umbrella and a jacket handy during those times of the year where the weather can change at the drop of a hat.

## Stress

To varying degrees, your body is constantly under stress. Whether it's trying to balance work and play or just trying to make it to that next pay check, you're experiencing stress. If you are in a career where you are constantly having to come up with ideas and meet deadlines, you are in a high-stress situation. Stress is one of the leading causes of the immune system being weakened.

There are many ways to manage and relieve stress. Choose an exercise routine that you like and can stick with to help you relieve it. Exercising can also jump start your immune system and keep your lymph nodes working properly. Reading, taking up a hobby, and even scheduling time to turn off all electronics can help with managing stress as well. Don't skip your off days. Take them. Use those days to decompress, have fun, or even go to a spa for a massage. If you have a family, plan an outing to a movie, a park, or just goofing off in the yard with them. Get your mind of your adult worries for a while.

## Chapter 2 - Antibiotics

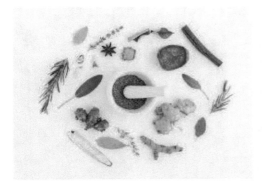

Since the discovery of penicillin, there have been over 100 types of antibiotics manufactured. Physicians often prescribe this type of medicine to fight bacterial infections. A problem is rapidly arising due to the over prescription of antibiotics, strains of bacteria that are resistant to the treatment. There is also a misconception of the use of antibiotics. These treatments so not fight nor do they eliminate viral or fungal infections.

The other problem with prescription antibiotics is they are not discriminatory as to what bacteria it attacks. The medicine also goes after the friendly bacteria in your small intestine, like Acidophilus and Bifidobacterium, two bacteria that aid in digestion and absorption of nutrients. Prescription antibiotics tend to kill bacteria of this type, often leading to yeast infections or other digestive issues.

There are herbals that can be used to fight bacterial infections. Herbal supplements will target just the infectious bacteria, leaving the friendly ones to do their jobs.

## Calendula *(calendula officinalis)*

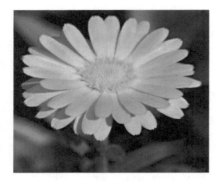

Better known as Marigold, this the petals of this flower have been known to fight topical infections and viruses as well.

## Cinnamon Stick *(cinnamomum zeylamcum)*

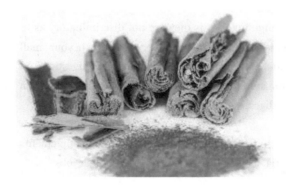

Yup, the seasoning we mostly use in desserts can also help fight bacterial infections. You can use it as the ground herb or even the essential oil.

**Dried Clove Bud *(syzygium aromaticum)***

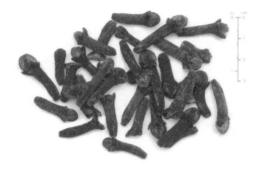

This seasoning is also a medicinal herb that can fight bacterial infections in the gut. You can also use this as an essential oil.

**Echinacea (echinacea angustifolia)**

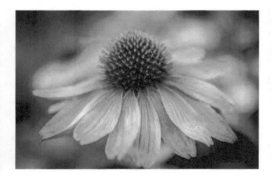

This is an herb that is highly effective in fighting infections and also speed healing from external injuries. Echinacea should be avoided if you have an auto-immune disease as it is an immune system booster.

### Garlic *(allium sativa)*

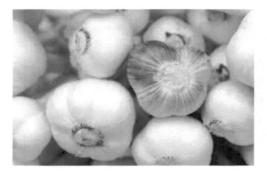

One of the kings in the herbal world, garlic can help to fight infectious bacteria, but due to the taste, most people just use it to cook with or chlorophyll coated tablets.

### Oregon Grape *(Mahonia aquifolium)*

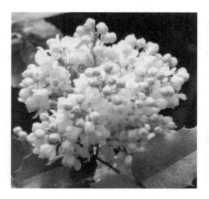

The root of this herb is highly potent in fighting bacterial infections. However, it should be passed by if you are pregnant, breastfeeding, diabetes, stroke, hypertension, or glaucoma.

### Usnea *(Usnea barbata)*

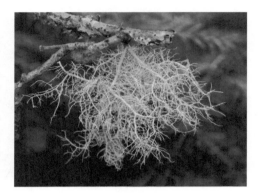

This is a natural, broad-spectrum antibiotic that is good for urinary tract infections, strep and staph infections, and other bacterial as well as fungal infections.

### Uva Ursi *(arcostaphylos uva-ursi)*

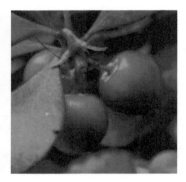

This herb is highly recommended for urinary tract infections. It should not be used for longer than two weeks, nor should it be administered to children, if you're nursing, or if you have kidney disease.

## Bergamot *(citrus bergamia)*

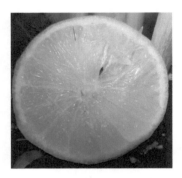

This essential oil is very good at killing bacteria related to urinary infections, meningitis and other infections. It has also been known to help in cases of shingles and chicken pox.

## Eucalyptus *(eucalyptus globulus)*

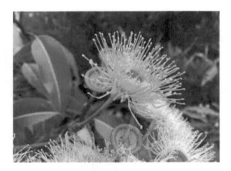

This essential oil is used topically to open airways and help to fight germs and infections. It can also be included blends for diffusers and sprays to sanitize surfaces to prevent further spread.

### Peppermint *(mentha piperita)*

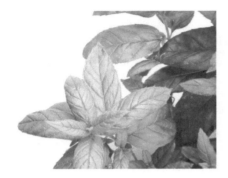

Peppermint essential oil is a highly effective disinfectant for bacteria, fungus, and other infections.

### Tea Tree Oil *(melaleuca alternifolia)*

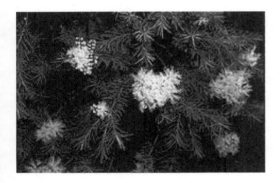

This highly antiseptic oil is great for fighting infections, both bacterial and viral. Studies have shown it is as just effective, if not more so, than bleach or disinfectant sprays.

## Antibiotic Syrup I

TOOLS NEEDED

Glass stock pot that holds three quarts or more of water
Strainer
Food scale
Bottle with lid large enough to hold a little over a quart of liquid
Wooden spoon
Funnel

INGREDIENTS

1/2 Ounce of Peppermint leaves
1/2 Ounce of Echinacea
1/2 Ounce of Calendula petals
1/2 Ounce of Cinnamon sticks
Quart of Purified water
2 Ounces of honey or glycerin

INSTRUCTIONS

- Bring the water to a boil
- Add the herbs
- Boil down to a pint
- Strain out the plant matter
- Place tea into the jar
- Add in honey or glycerin
- One tablespoon every few hours
- Stays good for up to a week in the refrigerator

**Antibiotic Syrup II**

INGREDIENTS

1/2 Ounce Oregon Grape root
1/4 Ounce Cloves
3/4 Ounce Peppermint leaves
1/2 Ounce Usnea
Quart of purified water
2 Ounces of honey or glycerin

Use the tools and instructions above.

**Salve I**

TOOLS NEEDED

Double boiler
Food scale
Jar with tight lid or more than one jar
Measuring cup
Wooden spoon
Funnel

INGREDIENTS

1 Cup Coconut Oil
1 Ounce beeswax
2 parts Calendula
1 Part Cinnamon stick
1 Part Echinacea
10 Drops Eucalyptus Essential oil
15 Drops Peppermint Essential oil

INSTRUCTIONS

- Place the wax and oil in a double boiler
- Add herbs once wax and oil has melted.
- Simmer for an hour
- Strain out herbs
- Place into jar
- Blend essential oils together
- Add the Essential oils when the salve is still warm but mixable.

**Salve II**

INGREDIENTS

1 Cup Coconut Oil
1 Ounce beeswax
2 parts Oregon Grape
1 Part Clove
1 Part Garlic
10 Drops Eucalyptus Essential oil
15 Drops Peppermint Essential oil

Follow instructions for tools and directions above.

**Antibiotic Tea I**

INGREDIENTS

1 tsp Echinacea
1 Cinnamon stick
1 tsp Calendula

## INSTRUCTIONS

- Boil the stick in 1 1/2 cups of purified water for 15 minutes
- Add the herbs to a cup
- Pour the water into a cup and cover to steep for 10 minutes
- Add honey to sweeten if needed.

**Antibiotic Tea I**

## INGREDIENTS

1/2 tsp cloves
1/2 Cinnamon stick
1 tsp Calendula petals
1/2 tsp Echinacea

## INSTRUCTIONS

- Boil the cinnamon and cloves in 1 1/2 cups of purified water
Follow the rest of the instructions above.

**Mineral Bath I**

## TOOLS NEEDED

1 large mixing bowl
1 small mixing bowl
Measuring cups
Mixing spoon
Storage container

INGREDIENTS

1 Cup of Magnesium Flakes

1/2 Cup of Sea Salt

1/2 Cup of Baking Soda

1/4 Cup Borax

1/2 Cup Calendula Petals

15 Drops of Peppermint Essential oil

15 Drops of Bergamot Essential oil

INSTRUCTIONS

- Mix the dry ingredients in one bowl and set aside
- Blend the essential oils in another bowl
- Add the dry ingredients to the essential oils
- Place in storage container overnight.
- Add 1/4 cup to running bath water

**Mineral Bath II**

INGREDIENTS

1 Cup Magnesium Flakes

1/2 Cup Sea Salt

1/4 Cup Oregon Grape Root, cut and sifted

1/4 Cup crushed cinnamon stick

10 drops Eucalyptus essential oil

15 drops Tea Tree essential oil

Follow the instructions for tools and mixing above.

## Chapter 3 - Immune System Boosters

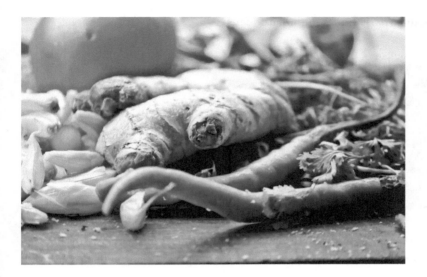

When discussing immune system boosters, you also have to include adaptogens. These herbs are "smart herbs" in that they do **double** duty. They help boost the immune system and strengthen the other body systems that are weak during illness. We have already listed some of the immune boosters **above**, but there are some we can add to the list.

## Astragalus *(astragalus membranaceus)*

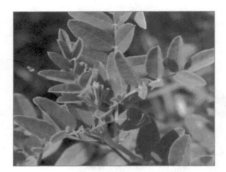

This is on the top of the list for adaptogens. Not only does this herb help to shore up the immune system, it also helps build blood and fights the fatigue that comes with contracting an illness.

## Elderberry *(sambucus nigra)*

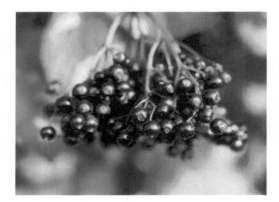

This herb has been known to improve immune system function, and when put into blends with antibiotics and antivirals can boost the action of the remedy.

### Ginger *(zingiber officinale)*

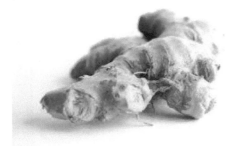

This herb has been used by itself and in blends for many centuries. It helps to boost the immune system and also acts as a catalyst for other herbs used with it. It is still used on its own today to reduce the severity and duration of a cold.

### Ginseng

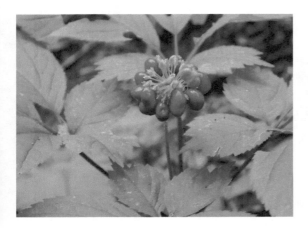

There are three types of this adaptogen with the Korean type being the most widely used. It helps to bring the body back into balance when its used by itself and helps to stimulate the immune system.

## Frankincense *(boswellia carteri)*

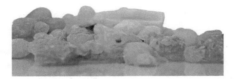

This essential oil is used as an immune booster, but it also has other benefits to help stimulate healing.

## Myrrh *(commiphora myrrha)*

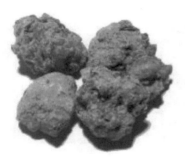

When added to a blend or other aromatherapy preparation, it helps to **protect** the immune system from further infection.

**Oregano *(organum vulgare)***

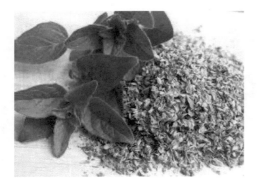

This immune booster is also used to combat bacterial and viral infections.

**Sage *(Salvia officinalis)***

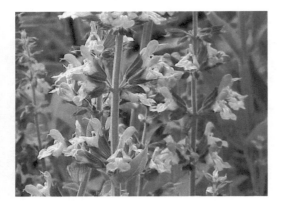

This all-purpose essential oil is especially recommended for the immune system, bacterial infections, viral infections, and fungal infections.

**Thyme Linalol *(thymus vulgaris)***

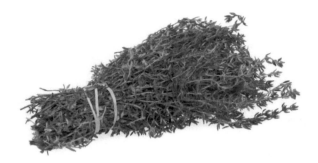

This essential oil boosts the immune system and also has antibacterial and anti-fungal properties.

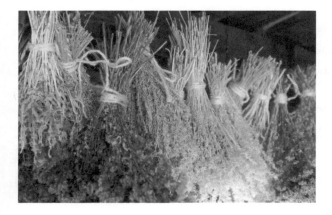

In this part of the chapter, I will be combing **herbs** and essential oils from the previous chapter. This is because too much of the **same** type of herb can lead to problems. Please, if you have any auto-immune **diseases,** do not include any herbs or essential oils that boost the immune system. They **can cause** flare-ups for your condition.

**Syrup I**

INGREDIENTS

1/2 Ounce of Elderberries
1/2 Ounce of Echinacea
1/2 Ounce of Peppermint Leaves
1/2 Ounce of Astragalus
2 Ounces of honey or glycerin
1 quart of purified water

(Instructions for tools and how to mix are in the previous chapter)

**Syrup II**

INGREDIENTS

1/2 Ounce Calendula Petals
1/4 Ounce of Cinnamon sticks
3/4 Ounce of Ginger
1/2 Ounce of Oregon Grape
2 Ounces honey or glycerin

**Lymph node rub I**

INGREDIENTS

4 Ounces of Sweet Almond Oil
15 Drops Frankincense essential oil
15 Drops Peppermint essential oil
10 Drops of Thyme Linalol

INSTRUCTIONS

- Mix all the ingredients together
- Pour into a dark colored squeeze bottle

Rub into the lymph node areas.

**Lymph node rub II**

INGREDIENTS

4 Ounces Sweet Almond oil
15 Drops Bergamot essential oil

15 drops Eucalyptus essential oil

10 Drops Sage essential oil

10 Drops Myrrh essential oil

(Instructions for tools and how to mix are in the previous chapter)

**Lymph node salve**

INGREDIENTS

1 Cup Coconut Oil

1 Ounce beeswax

2 parts Ginger

1 Part Elderberries

1 Part Astragalus

10 Drops Sage Essential oil

15 Drops Eucalyptus Essential oil

(Instructions for tools and how to make it are in the previous chapter)

**Chest salve**

INGREDIENTS

1 Cup Coconut Oil

1 Ounce beeswax

2 parts Cinnamon sticks

1 Part Ginger

1 Part Ginseng

10 Drops Oregano Essential oil

15 Drops Peppermint Essential oil

## Antibiotic/Immune Extract I

TOOLS NEEDED

1 quart-sized dark colored bottle with a tight lid

Food scale

Strainer

INGREDIENTS

1 Ounce of cinnamon sticks, crushed

1 Ounce of Calendula petals

1 Ounce of Astragalus

1 Ounce of Ginger

1 Pint of vinegar or alcohol

INSTRUCTIONS

- Place herbs in the bottle
- Add the liquid of your choice
- Shake the bottle twice a day for four days
- Strain out the herbs
- Add 15-20 drops of the extract to a beverage of your choice three times daily.

## Antibiotic/Immune Extract II

INGREDIENTS

1/2 Ounce of cloves

1 1/2 Ounce of Echinacea petals

1 Ounce of Ginseng

1 Ounce of Elderberries

1 Pint of vinegar or alcohol

**Immune booster bath I**

INGREDIENTS

1 Cup of Magnesium Flakes
1/2 Cup of Sea Salt
1/2 Cup of Baking Soda
1/4 Cup Borax
1/2 Cup Dried Ginger Slices
15 Drops of Eucalyptus essential oil
15 Drops of Sage Essential oil
(Instructions and tools are in the previous chapter)

**Immune Booster Bath II**

INGREDIENTS

1 Cup of Magnesium Flakes
1/2 Cup of Sea Salt
1/2 Cup of Baking Soda
1/4 Cup Borax
1/2 Cup Dried Elderberries
15 Drops of Bergamot essential oil
15 Drops of Frankincense Essential oil

**Immune Tea I**

1 tsp Calendula Petals
1 tsp Elderberries

**Immune Tea II**

1 tsp Ginger
1 tsp cinnamon

# Chapter 4 - Viruses

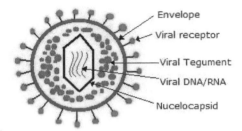

Envelope

Viral receptor

Viral Tegument

Viral DNA/RNA

Nucelocapsid

Colds, flu, pneumonia, and even HIV all have one thing in common. They are viruses. Viruses are organisms that can replicate in the system and attack certain parts of the body. It is due to this structure that antibiotics don't work, but like prescribed antibiotics, there are side-effects to prescribed antivirals. Here are a few alternatives.

*Herbal Supplements*

## Cat's Claw (*uncaria tomentosa*)

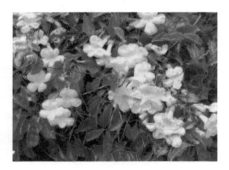

This rain forest herb has been highly recommended as an antiviral, antifungal, and an antibacterial. It has also been proven a more effective immune booster than Echinacea. Avoid if you are pregnant.

**Cranberry *(vaccinium macrocarpon)***

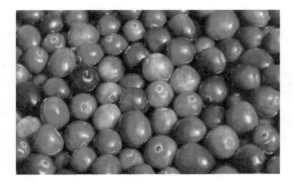

This little berry does have antiviral properties, but is better known for its ability to fight urinary tract infections.

**Lemon Balm Leaf *(melissa officinalis)***

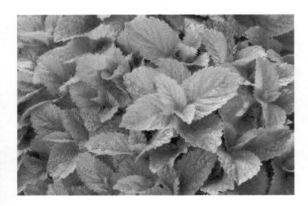

This herb has strong antiviral properties. Check with your doctor if you are pregnant.

### Licorice root *(glycyrrhiza glabra)*

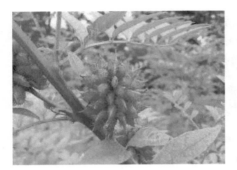

More famous for being made into candy, this root has strong antiviral properties and can kill H. pylori, a bacteria known for causing ulcers. It can cause diarrhea in large doses, and it is recommended that your not use it during pregnancy.

### Olive Leaf *(olea europaea)*

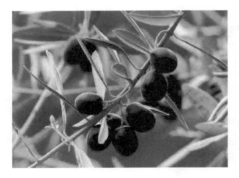

This herb comes highly recommended as an antiviral treatment for the flu or common cold. Take use it if you are pregnant.

### Lavender *(lavandula angustifolia)*

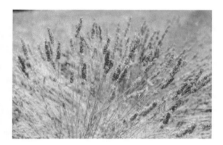

This essential oil is not only used for skin conditions, it is also known for its antiviral and immune boosting properties.

### Lemon *(citrus limon)*

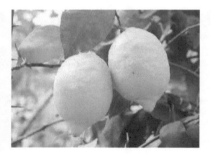

Lemon essential oil is highly potent when fighting viruses. It also helps to boost your immune system.

*Recipes*

## Viral Tea I

INGREDIENTS

1 tsp cranberries, dried
1 tsp ginger, dried
1 tsp Echinacea

## Viral Tea II

INGREDIENTS

1 tsp Olive Leaf
1 tsp Lemon Balm
1 tsp Cat's Claw

## Antiviral Rub I

INGREDIENTS

1 Cup Coconut Oil
1 Ounce beeswax
2 parts Elderberries
1 Part Olive Leaf
1 Part Ground Clove
10 Drops Eucalyptus Essential oil
15 Drops Lavender Essential oil

(Instructions for tools and how to make it are in Chapter 2)

**Antiviral Rub II**

INGREDIENTS

1 Cup Coconut Oil
1 Ounce beeswax
2 parts Cat's Claw
1 Part Echinacea
1 Part Lemon Balm
10 Drops Lavender Essential oil
10 Drops Peppermint Essential oil

(Instructions for tools and how to make it are in Chapter 2)

*Diffuser blends*

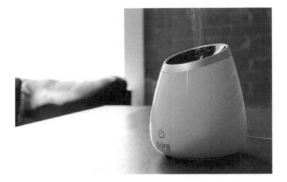

A diffuser is a machine that can heat undiluted essential oils in order to disperse an essential blend through a room. If you don't have a diffuser, you can use a candle warmer for the same effect.

**Antiviral Blend I**

INGREDIENTS

5 drops Lavender
5 Drops Thyme Linalol

**Antiviral Blend II**

INGREDIENTS

5 drops Eucalyptus
5 drops Lavender

**Antiviral Syrup I**

INGREDIENTS

1/2 Ounce Olive Leaf
1/2 Ounce Licorice
1/2 Ounce Echinacea
1/2 Ounce Elderberries
2 Ounces Honey glycerin
1 Quart purified water

(Tools needed and instructions can be found in chapter 2)

**Antiviral Syrup II**

INGREDIENTS

1/2 Ounce Olive Leaf
1/2 Ounce Licorice
1/2 Ounce Echinacea
1/2 Ounce Elderberries
2 Ounces Honey glycerin
1 Quart purified water

(Instructions and tools are in chapter 2)

**Antiviral bath I**

INGREDIENTS
1 Cup of Magnesium Flakes
1/2 Cup of Sea Salt

1/2 Cup of Baking Soda

1/4 Cup Borax

1/2 Cup Dried olive leaves

15 Drops of Lavender essential oil

7 Drops of Myrrh essential oil

8 Drops of Frankincense essential oil

(Instructions and tools are in chapter 2)

## Antiviral bath I

INGREDIENTS

1 Cup of Magnesium Flakes

1/2 Cup of Sea Salt

1/2 Cup of Baking Soda

1/4 Cup Borax

1/2 Cup Dried olive leaves

15 Drops Eucalyptus essential oil

5 Drops Thyme Linalol essential oil

5 Drops Sage essential oil

5 Drops Tea Tree oil

(Instructions and tools are in chapter 2)

## Chapter 5 - Cautions and Tips

There are a few thing you need to keep in mind when using and storing herbs and essential oils in your home.

*Herbal Storage*

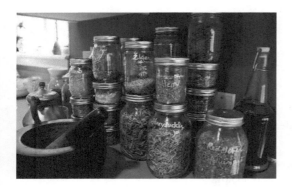

• Dried herbs can keep up to two years without losing their potency when stored in air-tight containers.

• Herbal Extracts have a shelf life of up to one year if stored in cool dry place.

• Herbal syrups store for up to seven days when you keep them in the refrigerator only four days on a shelf.

• Keep any herbal preparations away from children unless you are administering the remedy.

*Essential oil*

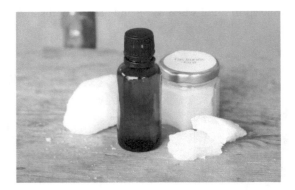

● Never use essential oils undiluted unless you are using them in a diffuser.

● Store essential oils in a cool dry place. Storing essential oils in a hot location in the house can cause them to evaporate in the bottle.

● Keep essential oils away from children.

● Salves keep for up to six months before they have to be tossed out.

*General information*

● Always look for all the information possible on any herbals and essential oils. There may be interactions with prescription drugs that have not been listed in this book.

● If you are ill, always visit your licensed physician for a proper diagnosis. I am not a physician.

Never stop looking up information on your new interest. There are websites out there that will give you good information. Here are a few:

https://www.aromaweb.com/
http://www.aromatherapy.com/
http://botanical.com/

Here are some recommended books:

*Today's Herbal Health*- Lousie Tenney, M.H.
*The Complete Book of Essential Oils & Aromatherapy*- Valerie Ann Worwood
*The Illustrated Encyclopedia of Essential Oils*- Julia Lawless
*The Way of Herbs*-Michael Tierra

There are also online groups and forums you can join for more information, recipes, and advice to continue coming up with new remedies, herbs, aromatherapy, and all things pertaining to natural health.

*Quick Tips*

• Chewing on a clove and swallowing the juice will help stop nausea.

• Peppermint essential oil on a cotton ball can provide relief from headaches.

• 2 drops of Lavender and 2 drops of Thyme Linalol on a damp wash cloth can be a quick boost to your immune system before you step out of the shower.

• Adding garlic to your soups can help boost your immune system and help fight infections.

• 15 drops of Tea Tree oil and 15 drops of Lemon essential oil in a spray bottle with purified water can sanitize surfaces.

• You can add cinnamon to any tea by stirring a stick in it.

• If you don't have lemon rind in your cooking, you can use drops of lemon essential instead. Just a few drops goes a long way.

• You can kill off lice in any shampoo by adding six drops of Tea Tree essential oil to one tablespoon of shampoo.

## Conclusion

In nature, there are many ways to heal the body and protect you from illness, but they can only be effective if you take care of yourself. It's easy to fall into bad habits, but there is a way to break them and put yourself on a path of health and wellness. Take small steps to make the transition into your new life.

I hope this books has helped you start your journey to being happier and healthier life, but don't stop with this book. A whole new world of natural health awaits you. Until next time.

Made in United States
Troutdale, OR
12/27/2023